Book 1
Nutrition

By: Bring On Fitness

&

Book 2
Weight Loss

By: Bring On Fitness

Book 1

Nutrition

The Beginners' Guide to Nutrition

By
Bring On Fitness

© Copyright 2018 – Bring On Fitness – All rights reserved.

The contents of this book may not be reproduced, duplicated, or transmitted without direct written permission from the author.

Under no circumstances will any legal responsibility or blame be held against the publisher for any reparation, damages, or monetary loss due to the information herein, either directly or indirectly.

Legal Notice:

Disclaimer Notice:

Please note the information contained in this document is for educational and entertainment purposes only. Every attempt has been made to provide accurate, up-to-date, complete, and reliable information. No warranties of any kind are expressed or implied. Readers acknowledge that the author is not engaging in the rendering of legal, financial, medical, or professional advice. The content of this book has been derived from various sources. Please consult a licensed professional before attempting any techniques outlined in this book.

By reading this document, the reader agrees that under no circumstances is the author responsible for any losses, direct or indirect, which are incurred as a result of the use of information contained within this document, including, but not limited to, errors, omissions, or inaccuracies.

About Bring On Fitness

Our passion for fitness gave life to **Bring On Fitness**. We started with the goal of helping as many people as we can. To educate, motivate and to help change peoples lives for the better. Bring On Fitness is not only for the fitness enthusiasts, but also for the beginner. We strongly believe nothing is more important than learning the basics and creating a strong foundation in both nutrition - through meal planning, and in exercise - by following a specific plan. This is just as important for the beginner, as it is for the experienced athlete.

We set high standards for ourselves, the information we share, and the products we carry. Our goal is to provide you with exceptional products that suit your needs and the knowledge and motivation to help you work towards and achieve your health and fitness goals.

Check us out at www.bringonfitness.com

"Our Mission is to have a positive impact in changing peoples lives. We will deliver the best possible fitness and nutrition solutions that will empower people to achieve their health and fitness goals."

Table of Contents

Introduction

Nutrition matters a lot – what you put in your body is what determines your health and even how you look. It doesn't matter if you're already fit or are just trying to lose weight; knowing what you're putting into your body and how it impacts you is essential to understanding your anatomy.

Nutrition is simply about eating the right foods and avoiding those that harm you in the long term. In this book, we're going to talk about what exactly are the different components in your food. We will look at how components, such as fats, carbs, and proteins, help your body and in what proportion should you eat them. You'll also get to know what kinds of food are the best sources for these macronutrients and what kinds of food you should avoid.

A whole chapter has been dedicated to studying calories – what calories are, how they react with your body, and what their function is. Calories are essential, especially from a weight loss point of view. If you have ever tried to lose weight, the first advice you will get is how to calculate your daily calorie needs. This book will give you a brief understanding of how calories determine your weight and how you can calculate your daily calorie needs.

We are also going to look at what good fats are and the importance of lean protein in your life. Lastly, we're going to focus on the different kinds of food and drinks that anybody who wishes to be healthy should avoid.

So, if you're looking for a book that helps you understand nutrition in detail and what you should eat and in what quantity, this is the book for you.

Chapter One: Overview of Nutrition

Our bodies are not simple, and they require a lot of nutrients to function properly. Our complex structure means that different kinds of nutrition fuel different parts of our body. So if you want to survive and function correctly, you have to work on your nutritional needs.

The composition of our diet can be divided into two major groups: macronutrients and micronutrients. Together, these make up most of our nutritional needs and help us survive.

Macronutrients

There are three macronutrients, and all of them perform a specific role in helping your body absorb energy. The only function that these three nutrients perform is supplying the body with energy, and this is why you need them in high amounts so that you can repair, develop, and grow.

The three macronutrients are carbohydrates, fats, and proteins. The best thing about macronutrients is that every food item that you eat will consist of at least one of these items. Even if it's a healthy snack bar or a raw vegetable, all kinds of food are made up of these nutrients.

Fats

Fats have a lot of stigmas attached to them and are considered to be harmful. In reality, you don't have to be scared of fats at all – they are an important part of any diet, and at least 15% to 20% of what you eat should have fats.

The main purpose of fats is that they help your brain to develop, enhance the functioning of your cells, protect different parts of your body (especially organs), and help your body absorb vitamins from the food that you eat.

As fats have more than twice the amount of calories as carbohydrates and protein, they are more difficult to burn off. Therefore, fats should be consumed sparingly.

The body breaks down fats into fatty acids, which are burned as energy. Fatty acids make a fantastic energy source for the body, although it is important to note that not all cells can use fatty acids for energy; brain cells, for example, do require glucose, so be careful when thinking about limiting your carbohydrate intake. If more fatty acids are broken down than the body needs for energy at that moment, then the fatty acids are packaged together in bundles called triglycerides and then stored in fat cells for use at a later date.

Some examples of healthy fats include olives, seeds (pumpkin, chia), avocados, almonds, and walnuts.

Protein

Proteins help your cells and body tissues regrow, and they also help repair them in case they are torn. You also need proteins to have a healthy immune system and achieve hormonal balance. Proteins also have amino acids, and these are essential for your body to release hormones. Out of the 20 amino acids that are found in proteins, nine are essential for the body.

Proteins are broken down into amino acids, which are used by the body to build new proteins. Each of these proteins has a specific function, such as enabling chemical reactions or allowing cells to communicate. If the body is low in glucose and fatty acids, then the body can get energy from protein, but this is not ideal.

The right sources of protein are seeds (hemp, flax, and chia), quinoa, avocados, beets, beans, pulses and legumes, raw greens (spinach and kale), and nuts (unsalted).

Carbohydrates

Carbohydrates consist of small sugar chains, which are broken down by your digestive system and converted into glucose – the body's primary source of energy. Carbohydrates should make up at least 45% to 65% of your food consumption.

Carbohydrates, when broken down by the body into glucose, are then absorbed through the walls of the small intestine. The liver processes the glucose. It then enters the body's circulatory system, increasing the body's blood glucose levels.

This provides the body with an excellent (and quickly accessed) source of energy. If there is excess glucose, the liver will store it to be used between mealtimes if the blood glucose levels fall below a certain level.

For individuals who are starting an active lifestyle and trying to lose weight, your carbohydrate intake should fall within 100 to 150 grams each day. The sources of carbohydrates should primarily be vegetables and fruit. You can also eat small amounts of healthy starches, such as sweet potatoes and potatoes (with the skin), as well as whole grains, such as brown rice and oats.

Many people wonder if fruits are healthy, as they are sweet and can add back fat to the body. In reality, fruit contains fructose, which is a more complex chemical than sucrose, which is present in sugar. So if your body is exposed to both, it will take more effort for it to digest the former than the latter. In the process, it ends up burning more fat from the body. So don't think eating fruit is bad for you, unless you are eating extremely sweet fruits all throughout the day. However, you might have to exercise precaution if you have high levels of sugar in your body.

Carbohydrates to choose: apples, carrots, oats, quinoa, chickpeas, brown rice, bananas, cauliflower, millet, and kidney beans.

Micronutrients

The body does not need micronutrients in the same amount as macronutrients, but that doesn't mean that they aren't important for the functioning of the body. Micronutrients complement macronutrients by working with them to keep the body moving and are essential to maintaining the right energy levels, cellular function, physical and mental well-being, and metabolism.

The two main micronutrients are vitamins and minerals.

Most people get their micronutrients from plants, which have a large amount of both vitamins and minerals. The amount of micronutrients in a plant depends on the soil that it was grown in. Micronutrients have a wide variety, from vitamin A, B, C, and K to minerals like zinc and magnesium, and all of them are essential for the body.

Chapter Two: Calories

Calories have received a somewhat negative reputation in recent decades, thanks to various fad diets and the tendency to discuss calories as unwanted things. In reality, calories are essential to our survival: if we do not eat enough calories on a daily basis, our bodies will not have the energy required to continue to function, and eventually, our bodies will break down.

All foods are a combination of three building blocks, and these are carbohydrates, proteins, and fats. The calories in each macronutrient are as follows:

- Carbohydrates – 4 calories

- Proteins – 4 calories

- Fats – 9 calories

Sugars, proteins, and fats are each broken down by the body into different compounds, which are then used by the body for different functions. Proteins, fats, and sugars each play an important role in the body, and it is essential to ensure that you are taking in enough of each so that your body has the energy and other resources that it needs to carry out all of its functions.

Calorie Needs

It is difficult to identify exactly how many calories our cells require to function properly, as each person's daily physical activities vary, along with his or her height, weight, age, and gender. To know approximately how many calories you need to consume per day so that you can achieve your weight loss goals, there are three crucial factors that you need to be aware of: Basal Metabolic Rate or BMR, Thermic Effect of Food, and Physical Activity.

These three factors need to be calculated, and by adding up the calculations from these, the result would be the total amount of calories required by your body each day. There are many calorie counters available online, all of which give different results based on the formulas they use. Adding the above three factors is the best and most accurate way to determine the amount of calories needed per day.

Here's a starting point for the number of calories you should be eating if you live a sedentary lifestyle.

For men (to maintain weight):

- Ages 19–30 should eat anywhere from 2,400 to 2,600.

- Ages 31–50 should eat anywhere from 2,200 to 2,400.

- Ages 51 and up should eat anywhere from 2,000 to 2,200.

For women (to maintain weight):

- Recommended: 1,600 to 2,000

Basal Metabolic Rate (BMR) – A person's BMR refers to the amount of energy required for his or her body to function while at rest, that is, for the lungs to continue breathing, the heart to keep pumping, the kidneys to keep functioning, and the body temperature to remain stable. These functions take up approximately 60% to 70% of the calories that are burned during the day. On average, the BMR of men is higher than that of women.

Age is an important factor in the formula because BMR tends to decline by 1% to 2% per decade after you turn 20, largely due to continued loss of fat-free mass in the body. This is, of course, a generalization, and it can differ among individuals depending on exercise, diet, and a person's percentage of body fat.

There are numerous formulas to calculate BMR, and they can be a little complicated. So you can use an online tool to calculate your BMR for you.

Physical Activity – After BMR, this is the second main factor that burns considerable amounts of calories. This includes all that you do with your body, such as walking to work, swimming at the pool, and talking to your friend. The amount of calories that are burned off from physical activity depends on your body weight. The more weight you have, the more calories you burn off as you engage in a particular physical activity. However, if you keep eating as many calories (if not more) as you burn off, you will continue to maintain your current weight (if not increase it).

A great tool to use to calculate how many calories each activity burns is at bitelog.com/exercise-search.htm, but many other online resources can help you to figure out how many calories you are burning.

While many people automatically think of activities like running or going to the gym as the best options for burning calories, there are many other activities that you can choose that will do a great job of burning calories. If you are one of those people, who prefer to disguise exercise in a fun activity; some of these options will work well for you.

Hiking and rock climbing are two excellent examples of fun, outdoor activities that will also help you burn a large number of calories. Depending on the difficulty of the trail and how quickly you are walking, you can burn around 400 calories per hour while hiking, whereas rock climbing can burn from 500 to 700 calories per hour. The difference in calories burned for rock climbing comes from how much you weigh because you are using your own body as the weight in this exercise. On days when the weather is not great, indoor rock climbing is always a great alternative.

If you have some household chores that need to get done and think you don't have time to exercise, think again: those chores are exercise! Vacuuming, laundry, sweeping, and mopping will all burn calories, and using those online resources mentioned earlier can help you figure out just how many calories each chore will burn. If you wash your car, it will burn about 200 calories per hour, and mowing the lawn (using a push mower, not a riding mower!) will burn around

300 calories per hour. Checking items off the "to-do list" and burning calories both make this option a great combination.

Playing sports is perhaps an obvious way to burn calories, but it still should be mentioned because it's a great way to have fun with your friends and still get your exercise in. Football can burn around 500 calories per hour, assuming that you and your friends are somewhat serious about the game, while soccer can burn 600 calories or even more per hour. Even badminton, which is a much lower impact sport, can burn between 250 and 400 calories depending on how much you weigh.

Thermic Effect of Food – This is the last factor that burns the calories that you consume, and it refers to the amount of energy that the body utilizes to digest the food that you have consumed. After all, it does take energy to digest the foods and then break them down into the basic organic compounds that the cells need to function properly.

To determine the number of calories that your body utilizes for this, what you do is multiply the total number of calories consumed within a day by 10%.

Chapter Three: Good Fats and Protein

Good Fats

Not all fats are bad for you; eating the right kind of fat will help you lose weight and build lean muscle, but remember that fat contains nine calories per gram, making it more than twice as dense as protein and carbohydrates (each of which has four calories per gram). Eating the right amount of healthy or good fats will help keep you feeling full longer, thus assisting in the weight loss process.

Your body also needs "healthy" fats to manage your mood, achieve top brain function, fight fatigue, and control weight. Your brain, for example, is almost 60% fat – this means that it needs fat to develop and function properly. These healthy fats can also help lower your cholesterol and the risk of heart disease, among other health benefits.

The "unhealthy" fats, on the other hand, can raise your risk of heart disease and increase your cholesterol, as well as cause a variety of other negative health outcomes. This is why it is essential to understand which fats are good and which are bad, as well as to focus on eating the ones that will help your body.

There are four main types of fat found in today's diet of foods developed from plants and animals: monounsaturated, polyunsaturated, trans fats, and saturated fats. Monounsaturated fats and polyunsaturated fats are considered to be the "good" fats, as they provide health benefits. Trans fats are definitively within the "bad" fats category, whereas saturated fats are still somewhat open to debate in the world of nutrition.

Omega-3 fatty acids are one of the most well known types of polyunsaturated fats, and they provide a phenomenal amount of health benefits. These benefits include: preventing and reducing symptoms of ADHD, depression, and bipolar disorder; preventing memory loss and dementia; reducing the risk of stroke, heart disease, and cancer; easing the symptoms of joint pain, arthritis, and inflammatory skin conditions; and supporting a healthy and viable pregnancy.

The best sources for omega-3s are fish, such as salmon, herring, anchovies, oysters, and lake trout. For those who are vegetarian or do not eat fish for other reasons, there are other options: algae, walnuts, Brussels sprouts, spinach, flaxseed, and kale, to name a few.

It is easy to distinguish the good fats from the bad or unhealthy ones. Overall, as indicated above, the "good" fats will be monounsaturated and polyunsaturated fats, which include omega-3s. However, other factors need to be considered when deciding on the specific foods that you will eat and determining whether they are providing good fats or bad fats.

In addition to trans fats, and possibly saturated fats, unhealthy fats are those that have undergone chemical alteration or processing, especially from plant-based fat sources. Meat or dairy fat sources that come from farm-raised animals or mass production are also unhealthy.

Protein

Protein is an essential macronutrient or building block that is known for repairing and creating muscle tissues. It is an essential part of fitness nutrition because it not only helps you lose weight but also promotes lean muscle growth. Now, when you hear the saying "lean protein," it refers to protein sources that have low fat content.

Aside from building lean muscle mass, eating lean protein also makes you feel full for longer periods of time, which in turn will minimize your food consumption and help you lose weight.

In reality, if you are eating the required minimum amount of calories per day, then you are most likely consuming enough protein. However, to build lean muscle mass, it is important to consider your sources of protein to ensure that this nutrient is coming with a well-balanced mixture of other nutritional elements.

Consuming protein helps your body burn more calories than fats or carbohydrates. Approximately 20% to 30% of the calories from proteins go toward the digestion process, while the range is between 5% and 15% for fats and carbohydrates. This is because protein is made up of amino acids, which are held by strong peptide bonds. Your body needs to be able to break down those bonds so that it can use the amino acids to repair tissues and to move oxygen through your bloodstream to form antibodies. To break those bonds, your digestion process has to work overtime, which ultimately results in it drawing more energy.

Remember, though, that just because you are getting more of your calories from protein instead of carbohydrates and fats does not mean that you can eat as many calories as you want. If you eat more calories, you will still gain weight, regardless of whether those calories are coming from protein or other sources.

The best time to eat protein is about 30 to 45 minutes after your workout, regardless of whether you were doing cardio activities or strength training. During that window, your muscles are particularly focused on rebuilding and on repairing the micro-tears that form when you work out. If you give your body protein, that rebuilding and repairing process will work even better, making you less sore the day after and improving your lean muscle mass.

To get the most out of the protein that you are eating, choose a snack that has 12 to 14 grams of protein with a calorie amount of around 40% of what you burned during your workout. So, for example, if you burned 300 calories on the elliptical, choose a snack that contains about 120 calories. Picking a snack that also contains some carbohydrates will help even more with muscle repair and energy replenishment.

The major sources of lean protein are the following: fish, soy, poultry, eggs, mushrooms, beef, beans, peas, lentils, seitan, and dairy. You will notice that there are both vegetarian and non-vegetarian options here, and just because you fall into one of these categories does not mean you cannot attain lean muscles. While meat, poultry, eggs, fish, and dairy do contain all nine amino acids that we get from food – which is why they are often referred to as "complete proteins" – it is very possible to get all of the amino acids from plant-based foods if you eat a balanced variety of such foods. So stop making excuses, and start doing all the right things for your body.

You need to keep in mind that having too much protein isn't a good thing, especially if you aren't working out. In fact, you only need between 40 and 50 grams of protein daily. If you aren't working out, this is a lot of protein and can do more harm than good. So, if you are working out, you need to make sure to get a good amount of protein in your system every day so you can effectively do your workouts. The protein will give you the energy you need to get through all the workouts and will keep you going beyond that.

Chapter Four: Foods to Avoid

Among the things that are proven unhealthy or even devastating in the long term, food is the first that comes to mind. Unhealthy food includes sugary drinks, pizzas, white bread, margarine, vegetable oils, pastries, cookies and cakes, French fries, ice cream, candy bars, processed meat, cheese, artificial sweeteners, and many others.

Sugary Drinks – If we were on a mission to find the unhealthiest product today, we would end up with added sugar. However, it must be emphasized that not all sources of sugar are bad. In the sea of unhealthy products full of sugar, the most important or the unhealthiest are sugary drinks. Many people don't realize that drinks also have calories and, because of that, they fail to understand that drinks can also be bad for health. Sugary drinks include sodas, fruit punches, lemonades, energy drinks, and other drinks with added sugar. Constant consumption of sugary drinks leads to obesity, which can have devastating effects on the human body. Surprisingly, fruit juices are also included in this category. Although they have more nutrients, they also contain very high levels of sugar and calories, which can be very easily neglected by people.

To avoid what was previously mentioned, people must abandon the practice of consuming sugary drinks and search for alternatives, such as water, soda water, tea, and many others. Among the drinks with the most sugar per ounce are the fruit juices, with a range of 4.75 to 7.15 grams of sugar per ounce, followed by regular sodas, energy drinks, iced tea, coffee, and sports drinks.

Pizzas – Pizza is the ultimate favorite food for so many of us. However, only a few of us understand the danger that pizza poses to our health. Similar to sugary drinks, pizza is also one of the reasons for the growing rate of obesity in the world. As regards the number of calories, 100 grams of pizza contain 266 calories, which is for sure a number you don't want to be a part of your daily eating habits. Aside from calories, some pizzas contain 1,620 mg of sodium and 33 grams of fat. One slice of cheese pizza also contains 5 grams of sugar.

However, not all pizzas are marked as unhealthy. To avoid the high intake of calories, fat, sugar, and other unhealthy nutrients, people often choose a vegetable pizza. Vegetable pizza contains vitamins A and C and more fiber in comparison to cheese or meat pizza. Add to this some veggie toppings, such as mushrooms, spinach, tomatoes, or onions, and you will get not only an amazing pizza but also a healthy intake of vitamins and other healthy nutrients.

White Bread – In the majority of cases, white bread is made of wheat, which contains gluten, and because of this, white bread is not good for people who are sensitive to gluten. However, white bread is bad not only for gluten-sensitive people but also for everybody else. White bread is mostly made of refined wheat, the healthy nutrients of which are reduced to a minimum because of the refining process. What you get in the end are pure calories, which can result in high blood pressure for some people. If you want to use bread, it is better to use whole grain bread instead of white bread. Whole grain bread contains a lot more vitamins, minerals, and fiber than white bread. All of this provides you with more energy throughout the day. One slice of white bread has 66 calories, 0.82 grams of fat, 12.65 grams of carbs, and 1.91 grams of protein. Yes, you do get some protein with white bread, but the damage the white bread is causing is much bigger than the benefits of the proteins it contains.

Specialty Coffee Drinks – Fancy coffee drinks with a variety of delicious flavorings are a popular option for many people, but unfortunately, these drinks tend to be extremely high in calories. The problems with these coffee drinks are the same as those with sugary drinks discussed above: empty calories and little, if any, nutritional value. Moreover, we tend to add sugar (or artificial sweeteners) and milk or cream to these drinks, increasing the caloric content even further.

Plain black coffee can help with weight loss because caffeine will boost your metabolism. Adding low fat or part-skim milk is fine, but try to avoid adding sugar or sweeteners.

Processed Meat – Unlike unprocessed meat, processed meat is proven to have negative effects on your health. Several studies around the world indicated that some serious diseases, such as colon cancer, diabetes, and heart disease, could be the result of the consumption of processed meat. If we were to look for a definition of processed meat, it would be that processed meat refers to meat that has been cured, salted, dried, canned, and smoked. In the category of processed meat, we can include hotdogs, sausages, salami, bacon, and ham.

According to some studies, processed meat contains N-nitroso compounds that are proven to be cancer-causing elements. The most important thing about the intake of processed meat is self-control. You must be able to determine the maximum amount of processed meat you are going to eat and decide on what type of processed meat you will be eating because not all types of processed meat are equally unhealthy.

Conclusion

Nutrition is not as simple as just learning about things. You have to apply your knowledge to your everyday routine and make sure that you genuinely change your lifestyle to include things that are better for your health.

Before you make any substantial changes regarding what you eat, you should consult your doctor. This is important just to make sure that you all your nutritional requirements are being met.

More importantly, to attain a healthier lifestyle, you need to motivate yourself to do better. You can keep a diary where you can record all the positive changes in your life or something like a before/after picture. These little things will help push you to cut out all the unhealthy food from your life.

Make sure that you have your friends and family supporting you throughout this process.

Thank you, and remember to share how well these meal planning and organization tips work for you. You can do that by writing a review in your Amazon account under Your Orders.

Thank you,

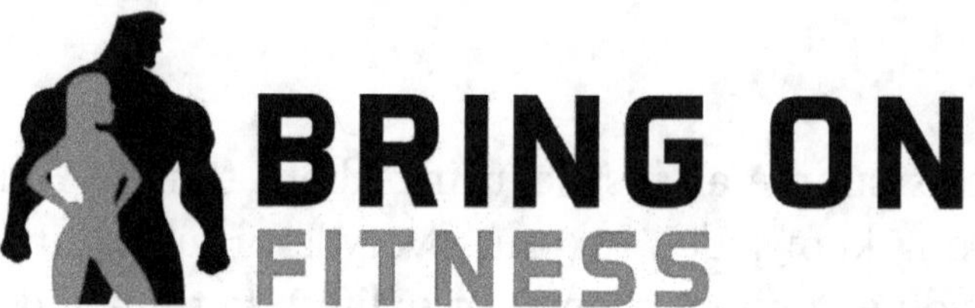

Resources

http://www.eatright.org/resources/food/nutrition

https://www.bornfitness.com/fix-your-diet-understanding-proteins-carbs-and-fats/

https://www.medicalnewstoday.com/articles/263028.php

https://www.nhs.uk/Livewell/loseweight/Pages/understanding-calories.aspx

Book 2
Weight Loss

20 Reasons Why You Are Not Losing Weight

By
Bring on Fitness

About Bring On Fitness

Our passion for fitness gave life to **Bring On Fitness**. We started with the goal of helping as many people as we can. To educate, motivate and to help change peoples lives for the better. Bring On Fitness is not only for the fitness enthusiasts, but also for the beginner. We strongly believe nothing is more important than learning the basics and creating a strong foundation in both nutrition - through meal planning, and in exercise - by following a specific plan. This is just as important for the beginner, as it is for the experienced athlete.

We set high standards for ourselves, the information we share, and the products we carry. Our goal is to provide you with exceptional products that suit your needs and the knowledge and motivation to help you work towards and achieve your health and fitness goals.

Check us out at www.bringonfitness.com

"Our Mission is to have a positive impact in changing peoples lives. We will deliver the best possible fitness and nutrition solutions that will empower people to achieve their health and fitness goals."

Table of Contents

Introduction

You cannot stand in line at the supermarket or flip through television channels without seeing people celebrated for their thin, attractive bodies. Some people have worked hard to maintain their physique, while others rely on Photoshop and other techniques to make them appear thinner.

Regardless, it puts a lot of pressure on people to lose weight. This can be seen in crazes over weight loss fads, including workout plans, diets, and miracle supplements that are intended to help us lose weight quickly. There is such an obsession with looking great that there is a huge market for the weight loss industry and plenty of ways for companies to capitalize on the desires of others. In America alone, nearly $60 billion is spent on weight loss methods, including low-calorie foods, bariatric surgery, diet pills, health club memberships, and much more.

The downside of all this money spent is that it is not always effective. In fact, many people who lose weight fail to keep it off. Others try to lose weight and plateau, hitting a standstill before they come close to their weight loss goal. So when it seems like you have tried everything, what do you do?

The truth of the matter is that there are many reasons you may not be losing the weight that you want. Some have to do with your diet, while others have to do with the methods you are using to meet your weight loss goals. The good news is that by learning more about your body and the science behind how it works, you can both achieve and maintain your weight loss.

When it comes to weight loss, there is no such thing as starting tomorrow. Start right now by reading through the pages of this book. By the end, you will have some insight into the reasons why you are having trouble losing weight.

Mistake #1: Your Training Regime is Predictable

One common message for people trying to lose weight is that they should move around more. Even doing small things like walking around more at work, parking further away from the entrance of places of business, and taking the stairs instead of the elevator has been proven to help people increase the number of calories they are burning, thus causing weight loss. However, more recent studies show that there is a maximum point for calorie expenditure. This means that, at some point, even with intense exercise, your body stops burning calories. This means that you could be doing extra work for nothing.

According to the NYU Langone Medical Center Medical Weight Management Program director, Holly Lofton, it is quite common for people who pair extreme workouts with the same dietary habits to plateau with weight loss. It may work at first, especially for those who live a more sedentary lifestyle, but eventually, weight loss comes to a halt.

One thing that you can do to combat this problem is to switch up your workout routine. If you rely on biking or walking to lose weight, try swimming or yoga instead. You can also learn more about your body by finding out at what point you plateau. Each body reacts differently to exercise. For example, someone with a higher body fat percentage is more likely to burn more calories before plateauing than someone with a lower body fat percentage. Factors like muscle mass, genetic markers, metabolism, and hormone levels can also affect how many calories you can burn before reaching that plateau.

Mistake #2: Your Body Cannot Put More Calories Out without Storing Some

Even though evolution has changed the human body in many ways, many of our primitive instincts and patterns still exist. One of these primitive instincts is to survive by ensuring the body has enough calories to perform its regular functions. Associate Professor of Anthropology Herman Pontzer worked with his associates on a study that examined the way the body uses a system of checks and balances to ensure survival when it comes to burning calories.

The study examined people with sedentary lifestyles compared to hunter-gatherer populations in Tanzania. The conclusion was that even though the Tanzanian hunter-gatherers are incredibly active, with the men walking 10 miles per day and the women walking 6 miles, they do not expend more calories than a more sedentary person.

This phenomenon can be explained by dividing calories into two categories—resting calories and activity calories. The resting calories are those that the body stores to ensure that it is functioning in the way it is supposed to. This is necessary to fight against inflammation, keep the immune system healthy, and ensure the body is receiving and responding to signals from the brain. These resting calories are necessary for health.

Outside of the resting calories are the activity calories, which are those that are freed up so they can be burned during physical activity. Once you run out of the activity calories, your body will burn rest calories—but only at a very slow rate. This is a primitive function that ensures health. After all, it does no good to lose weight if your immune system is not functioning properly and you get sick.

Mistake #3: You Are Stressed Out

For a long time, the latest dieting trends were all you heard about for weight loss. Things like restricted-calorie eating, the cabbage soup diet, and other trends could produce results—but only to an extent. Plus, the statistics do not lie. The majority of people who can lose weight with a diet end up gaining that weight back (and often, more weight than they started with) within five years. This is proven by several studies, including one in 2002 that analyzed 231 million dieting Europeans—only 1% were able to attain permanent weight loss following their diet.

One of the reasons that dieting is next to impossible (and ineffective) is because of the stress it causes. Stress is the enemy of dieting for two reasons. First, it increases the body's production of the hormone cortisol. Cortisol is known for causing the body to store fat poorly, especially around the abdominal area.

Additionally, stress is more likely to cause binge eating. This can make you sit down and eat more calories than your body needs—and then store it, as a result. This is incredibly detrimental to weight loss efforts. In this case, it would seem that making lifestyle changes, rather than sticking to a diet, would be a better option for losing weight.

Mistake #4: Metabolic Suppression

One of the most popular shows for weight loss miracles is "The Biggest Loser"—a competition in which the contestants' goal is to lose weight. On average, the contestants lose 129 pounds each. Unfortunately, a study done six years later found that the participants had gained back an average of 70% of the weight they had lost. Additionally, they were burning fewer calories than the average person of their weight and size—about 500 calories less, to be exact.

This study mirrors similar studies that have examined the weight regulation in the mind. This is known as a set point. Basically, each person has a set point for their weight, which their body tries to maintain. When you drop below your body's set point, the mind starts to fight back against dieting.

The brain fights back in a few ways. First, it reduces the number of calories burned during physical activity compared to the calories burned for the average person. This is known as metabolic suppression because the brain is suppressing how quickly the metabolism works. Second, it affects the way you eat. Not only does it produce hunger hormones to encourage you to eat more, it lights up the pleasure center in your brain, such that eating becomes more rewarding.

Mistake #5: You Are Depriving Yourself

Studies done with rats show how food deprivation affects the mind. One study restricted the amount of food that rats were allowed to eat for five days and then gave them unlimited Oreos for two days. This was done for several weeks. Then, a stressor was introduced to the rats with the restricted diet and a control group. The study showed that the rats who were dieting ate twice as many Oreos following exposure to the stressor when compared with the control group. Then, it was noted that even when a single bite of Oreo was eaten, the rats would binge on regular food when it was available.

One of the reasons why diets do not work is because a diet encourages the deprivation mindset. When the body and mind are deprived, whether through calorie restriction or drastic diet changes, it changes the way that neurotransmitters like dopamine work in the brain. It makes eating more pleasurable and causes you to seek out unhealthy foods as a result, to experience this reward.

The same study has also shown that once the dieting period was over, binge eating was still a problem. This may explain why, following a successful diet, people are still likely to gain the weight back. Instead of depriving yourself, consider having a cheat meal. Do not make it a whole day where you binge eat, but know that it is okay to give into your cravings on occasion.

Mistake #6: You Are Eating Too Much

Often, people eat not because they are hungry, but because external cues are telling them that they need the food. The food marketing industry is partly to blame for this, particularly the problem of overeating. It is harder to resist something when you are getting a deal. For example, why get a half-size sub when you can get a full one for just a dollar or two more? When it is only a dollar to supersize a meal and get more food (and more calories), it just seems to make sense to get the larger amount of food. Food selling techniques have also become extreme—with companies even using sexuality to sell things like burgers.

Another problem is falling into negative habits with your food. Imagine that a couple of nights out of the week, you eat a snack and watch television right before bed. This is a poor choice simply because you are eating calories right before you go into a restful state for the night. However, if done regularly, you may find yourself craving snacks just because you are sitting down in front of the television. This leads to eating even when you are not hungry.

The key to overcoming this is learning to eat when you are actually hungry, rather than whenever the thought crosses your mind. Pay attention to physical body cues that indicate you are hungry, like a growling stomach or fatigue that indicates a need to refuel. Then, eat at a slow enough pace that you can register when you start to feel full—and stop eating.

Mistake #7: You Have Trouble Detecting Hunger/Fullness Cues

Many people who have trouble overeating struggle with understanding their own bodies. They may have been used to eating whatever they want whenever they feel like it for so long that they cannot even tell when they are hungry or full. This is a problem because it often leads to eating more food than you need to consume. These extra calories translate to stored fat.

One of the best ways to learn to listen to your body is to start eating in an area that is free of distractions. If this does not work, there may be emotional reasons or an underlying problem that drives you to eat. Discovering this can help you find the root of your problematic relationship with food.

Another technique that you can use is putting smaller portions on your plate. Given that your desire to avoid waste sometimes overwhelms feelings of fullness, making you feel like you must clean your plate, it is better to eat smaller portions.

When you cannot detect the cues at all, the best answer may be eating on a set schedule. Eat a small snack two to three times per day, and eat a meal three times daily. Ideally, you should speak with a nutritionist about the ideal calorie range for someone of your weight who wants to lose weight. Then, fit your meals into this calorie range.

Mistake #8: You Aren't Slowing Down to Eat

Did you know that your body is satisfied with food long before your mind is? While eating nourishes your physical body, it has effects on the mind as well. One of the biggest mistakes that people make is trying to eat their food quickly. This is problematic because it takes time for the food to pass from mouth to stomach and even longer for the brain to register that the body is full.

To overcome this problem, you must start slowing down when you eat. Fully chew each bite, and take a few breaths before going for another one. Pay attention to how your stomach feels as you eat. Once you have fulfilled your needs, you will notice that you are not enjoying the food as much. You may also feel pressure in your stomach. If you overeat, it can cause discomfort, pain, or queasiness. Overeating can also affect your body later on, as it slows down to process your full stomach.

Ideally, by slowly and thoughtfully chewing each bite, you will learn to stop eating when you are full. Many people eat more than their bodies need, and this can make it nearly impossible to lose weight—even when making healthier food choices.

Mistake #9: Your Hunger Cues Are Being Confused with Something Else

Hunger cues are not the only thing that drives you to eat. There are several other triggers that people experience, which can be confused as a signal from the body that you are hungry. These include:

- Mind Hunger – If you develop excessive eating habits, like eating a certain amount of food simply because it is "time" to eat, it can cause you to think you are hungry when you are not.
- Teeth Hunger – Sometimes, the urge to have a cigarette or chew on something comes to you in times of frustration. You are not hungry, but you have an oral fixation that needs to be satisfied. Try chewing a piece of gum instead.
- Mouth Hunger – The smell or sight of food has the potential to make your mouth water and feel hungry, which can bring about cravings unrelated to hunger.
- Emotional Hunger – Food can be pleasurable and even comforting. This is what causes emotional eating in some cases, which is often a result of filling a void by using food or using it to push your feelings down.
- Fatigue – If you are overly tired, lack of food may not be to blame. It can also result from not getting enough sleep or working too hard.
- Thirst – Being thirsty can cause you to feel hungry, often because of the sluggishness that results from dehydration. Try drinking a glass of water when you think you are hungry before you try eating.

Mistake #10: You Are Only Focusing on the Numbers

Often, people who are trying to lose weight are aiming to see a certain number on the scale. The problem is that weight loss does not always result in lower numbers, especially for people who are building muscle tone through exercise during their efforts. This happens because muscle weighs more than fat, so gains in muscle can actually appear as if you are increasing in weight instead of losing it.

There are also other factors that affect weight loss. These include things like water weight, how quickly the foods you are eating are digested, and your bowel movements. If you want a more accurate measurement, consider using how you look and how clothes fit as indicators that you are moving in the right direction.

It is important to remember that weight loss is not so much about hitting a certain number as it is about becoming healthier and improving your fat-to-muscle ratio. Do not focus on the numbers—focus on the results.

Mistake #11: You're Making Efforts, but You Are Not Tracking Them

Many people consume more calories each day than they think—even hundreds more. It is true that making small changes to your diet and lifestyle, such as moving around more and making healthier eating choices, can help with weight loss efforts. If you are not tracking what is happening, however, you may not be doing enough.

In today's age of technology, it is easier than ever to track your calories and activity. There are countless apps and devices designed to help make losing weight significantly easier. Some devices may track calories burned or how far you walk, while others measure sleep patterns and heart rate, too. Even calorie counting apps can be sophisticated, letting you scan bar codes of the foods you eat or input food items to calculate your total caloric intake.

The apps and devices that you choose to work with are ultimately up to you. Keep in mind, however, that by knowing what is working and what isn't, you can drastically improve your efforts.

Mistake #12: You Think That Healthy Foods Have No Calories

When you are trying to lose weight for better health, keep in mind that it is not always the numbers that matter. For your body's metabolism to stay at a healthy rate and for you to diet without feeling hungry, you should seek foods that are wholesome in nature.

Did you know that many diet foods contain processed ingredients that are not-so-healthy for your body? They may be low in calories, but they are also low in nutrition. For example, diet sodas are a popular choice for people looking for a low-calorie soda alternative. However, diet soda has actually been seen to increase people's weight in a few studies, although science is still out on the reasoning behind this.

Instead of seeking out these foods, opt for more wholesome foods. Eat a diet rich in protein, whole grains, and fruits and vegetables. When you are making food choices, do not count calories—make your calories count.

Mistake #13: You Are Not Eating Enough Protein

One of the most important foods for a person who is trying to lose weight is protein. Protein has numerous benefits for people trying to lose weight. One of the first things to note is that when you pay attention to your body cues and eat when you are hungry, protein can stave off hunger. This is because the body digests it slower, so it stays in your stomach longer. Protein consumption also boosts metabolism. Finally, the way that protein affects the brain can also increase weight loss.

High levels of protein can alter the hormones produced by the area of the brain known as the hypothalamus. It is the hypothalamus that helps regulate weight. When you consume higher amounts of protein and reduce fat and carbs, it reduces the production of the hunger hormone and increases the production of satiety hormones that tell your body it is full. This means you may eat fewer calories. For most diets, it is recommended that around 30% of your daily caloric intake should come from protein.

The quality of the protein you are eating can also affect how quickly you are losing weight. Consider lean meats for protein, such as fish, chicken, and hamburger with a lower fat content. Whole grains and beans are other good, wholesome sources of protein.

Mistake #14: You're Skipping Out on the Weights

Many people know the importance of trying to be more active when trying to lose weight, but did you know that regular muscle workouts are an important part of losing and maintaining weight loss? The body is not always picky about what it is burning. If you are not using your muscles regularly, you may find that your dieting regimen is causing you to lose muscle mass in addition to fat. This is because the body will burn this up to make up the reduction in calories, too, especially if you are not working out.

You also will find that you look better once you have lost weight if you continue to tone your muscles. It can help reduce the amount of extra skin that is left behind once you lose weight. Additionally, lifting weights can help keep your metabolism working how it is supposed to, preventing the slow down that can bring your weight loss efforts to a screeching halt.

You do not have to strain yourself to lift weights. Start with a few repetitions of a low weight, even if it is just 10 or 15 pounds. As you increase the weight you are lifting, you will burn more calories and improve the way you look.

Mistake #15: You Are Doing Too Much Low-Intensity Cardio Training

When you are trying to lose weight and get healthier, cardiovascular workouts can speed up your progress. Some workouts, such as jogging and running, have received bad publicity in the last few years because of their impact on joint health, but there are plenty of alternatives that can get your heart pumping fast. This includes swimming, jumping on a trampoline, and using an elliptical machine.

In the past few years, one type of exercise that has received a lot of hype for burning fat is high-intensity interval training or HIIT. During this type of exercise, you keep a steady pace and then you work to increase your heart rate for a set period of time. Then, you take another small break, but keep moving. For example, you would jog for five minutes and then run for two, followed by another period of jogging.

In general, cardiovascular exercise is a critical part of weight loss. It helps burn belly fat, which can be stubborn to get rid of. It also offers numeral health benefits, including reducing your risk of heart disease and eliminating visceral fat, which builds up around the organs.

Mistake #16: You Are Not Sleeping Enough

Studies show that individuals with poor sleeping habits are more likely to be obese. These statistics show a 55% greater risk for adults and an 89% greater risk for children. A study conducted by the University of Chicago uncovered the reason behind this correlation—"metabolic grogginess."

When you do not get enough sleep, the fat cells in your body feel the deprivation. The result is difficulty using insulin, which can lead to insulin encouraging fat storage in your body. This can even cause insulin resistance, storage of fat in the liver, and diabetes.

Additionally, a lack of sleep upsets the balance of leptin and ghrelin. Leptin is responsible for telling you when you are full, which means you feel hungry even when you are not. Ghrelin stimulates hunger and reduces hormones in excess, and a lack of sleep encourages its production.

Additionally, not getting enough sleep can affect the frontal lobe, which is responsible for decision making. This can leave you more susceptible to poor dieting choices because it becomes increasingly hard to resist the temptation.

Mistake #17: You Aren't Choosing the Right Diet for Your Body

One of the problems with fad diets is that they treat everyone as the same rather than as the individual that they are. For example, some people respond well to a reduced-calorie diet, while others cut out fat and are successful. However, not everyone's body is built the same way. For some people, low-carbohydrate diets are the best option.

One variation of low-carb diets is a Ketogenic diet, where you increase protein and fat intake while reducing carbohydrates almost completely. Some studies have shown that in the short term, these diets cause as much as two to three times the amount of weight loss as a typical low-fat diet. Additionally, low-carb diets can improve good cholesterol levels, manage blood sugar, and improve triglycerides.

Ideally, the diet you choose should reflect factors like your metabolism and what your problem areas are. This will help you find the diet that is most effective. Additionally, keep in mind that many diets have additional health benefits, not just weight loss. Consider what will help you the most, and adjust as needed until you see the results that you want.

Finally, be patient with the results. You often cannot tell if a diet is working for several weeks because of the numerous factors that cause weight to fluctuate.

Mistake #18: You Are Drinking Too Much

It is not always the food that we are putting in our bodies that is the problem when it comes to weight loss. Even supposedly healthy drinks, such as vitamin beverages and juices, are high in sugar, which can contribute to an increased caloric intake. This is problematic because beverages are not filling. This means that you are taking in these extra carbohydrates and still craving food. These drinks are okay in moderation, but too much can be problematic.

The amount of water you drink can also affect how much weight you are gaining or losing. When you drink water, it has been proven that the number of calories you burn can be boosted for the next hour and a half by an impressive 24% to 30%. Another study showed that drinking about two cups (17 ounces) of water about half an hour prior to a meal increased weight loss by 44%. This means that if you are dieting, drinking water can drastically boost the results you are seeing.

Alcohol can be another problem beverage for weight loss. Beers and some types of sugary liquors have high sugar content that can add unnecessary calories. Additionally, most alcohols contain seven calories per gram of liquid. This does not mean that you have to quit completely, but try to drink only moderate amounts of alcohol. You should also stick to vodka and other spirits, mixed with a beverage that does not have calories.

Mistake #19: You Are Trying to Lose Too Much Too Fast

People who are trying to lose weight often want to see results fast. The problem with this is that rapid weight loss is not healthy for the body. It is also nearly impossible to maintain if you go back to a normal or less intense diet and exercise regimen.

The best way to lose weight is gradually. The people who are most effective at maintaining their weight loss may lose just 1 to 2 pounds of weight each week or less.

Something else to keep in mind regarding expectations is that there are external factors that can influence weight gain. For example, having conditions like PCOS, diabetes, hyperthyroidism, or sleep apnea can cause weight gain. There are also many medications for treating different conditions that can cause the person taking them to gain weight. If you believe that an underlying condition or a medication may be the root of your struggles in losing weight, consult with your physician about the best route for you to take.

Mistake #20: Your Body Needs a Break

Constant dieting is not healthy. Additionally, when you diet for a long period of time, you may find that you start gaining back weight the moment you decide to try and manage your weight rather than losing it. This has a lot to do with the body's set point, which can be lowered—but must be lowered gradually to be effective.

Sometimes, the best thing to do when you plateau with weight loss is not to fight back harder by reducing calories more or increasing your workout. Instead, try taking a break from weight loss, and work to maintain that weight. By maintaining a lower weight, you will help adjust your body's weight set point.

Ideally, you should take a break and try to maintain that lower weight for one to two months before starting another diet and exercise regimen. During this time, make sure you are getting plenty of sleep and still working to build lean muscle. By doing this, you are encouraging your overall health and ensuring that you maintain your weight loss instead of gaining it back, as many people do.

Conclusion

When you are trying to lose weight, there are many factors fighting against you. Fortunately, knowledge is half the battle when it comes to understanding your body and why you may not be losing weight. Take a good look at your weight loss efforts, and compare them against the information you have read so far. Chances are you will find the reason or reasons why you have not been successful.

The good news is that it is never too late to start working toward a healthier, happier, and fitter you. Take your new knowledge, and use it to help you lose weight in a way that works. Learn to listen to your body—you can often tell by the way that it feels what it needs.

Thank you, and remember to share how well these weight loss tips work for you. You can do that by writing a review in your Amazon account under Your Orders.

Thank you,

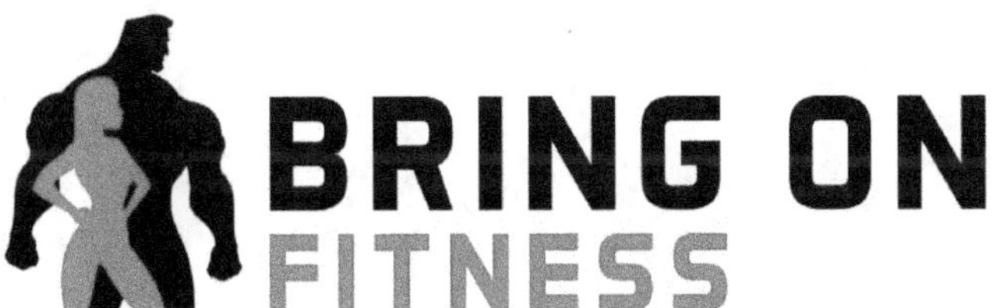

References

http://www.fitnessforweightloss.com/diet-and-weight-loss-statistics/

https://www.cnn.com/2016/01/28/health/weight-loss-exercise-plateau/index.html

https://www.nytimes.com/2016/05/08/opinion/sunday/why-you-cant-lose-weight-on-a-diet.html

http://www.findingbalance.com/articles/understanding-hunger-and-fullness-cues/

https://www.healthline.com/nutrition/how-protein-can-help-you-lose-weight

https://www.healthline.com/nutrition/20-reasons-you-are-not-losing-weight#section3

https://www.cbsnews.com/news/can-diet-soda-make-you-gain-weight/

https://www.shape.com/lifestyle/mind-and-body/why-sleep-no-1-most-important-thing-better-body